Table of Contents

Introduction

Multiple deployment cycles to Iraq and Afghanistan combat zones and the increase in Post-Traumatic Stress Disorder (PTSD) have resulted in new challenges for Army leaders.[1] PTSD is defined as "an anxiety disorder that can develop after exposure to a life threatening event or witness to such event and can cause cognitive, physical, and emotional alteration to individuals."[2] However, PTSD is not a new phenomenon in the military but has been called several different names throughout history – irritable heart, shell shock, combat exhaustion, war neurosis, combat stress, and combat fatigue. Emotional responses and behavioral reactions to life-threatening experiences have likely occurred since humans hunted animals and competed with other humans for survival.[3] As humans began to live collectively, warfare inflicted physical and mental trauma on participants, becoming an innate component of the human response. Throughout history, commanders of military units have ignored, suppressed, or taken measures to manage the natural responses to human conflict.

The responses of military leaders and society to military men and women impaired by trauma such as PTSD have varied throughout American history.[4] During the American Revolutionary War (1775-1783), General George Washington built and maintained a regular Army to face the British Empire. Washington's porous formation was comprised of men who lacked the reliability to face combat for an unknown period of time.[5] In addition to the superior

---

[1] Robert D. Haycock, "A Time for Change: Attacking the Stressors Vice the Symptoms" (Monograph, U.S. Army Command and General Staff College, 2009), 4.

[2] American Psychiatric Association, *Diagnostic and Statistical Manual of Mental Disorders*, (Washington, D.C. 1980), 213.

[3] F. Don Nidiffer and Spencer Leach, "To Hell and Back: Evolution of Combat-Related Post Traumatic Stress Disorder," *Developments of Mental Health Law* 29 (2010): 1-23.

[4] Ibid., 13.

[5] Ibid., 14.

capabilities of the British ground and sea campaign, high rates of desertion, low morale, and lack of funding from the fledgling government were the operating conditions General Washington faced.[6] Strict discipline was critical to Washington's leadership style, and at that time, little effort was expended to understand the effects of combat. Punishment for mental health problems and desertion was harsh and included flogging, running the gauntlet, tar and feathering, and shackles. Offenders might find themselves placed in a cage complete with wooden spikes, which was moved by a horse.[7] Over the course of the war, General Washington lobbied Congress to issue over 700 execution orders for crimes.[8] The intent of the punishment was to deter other soldiers from committing the same act and to persuade them to formations.

Not all public figures supported General Washington's treatment of soldiers. Dr. Benjamin Rush, a signer of the Declaration of Independence and recognized as the father of American psychiatry, suggested that soldiers suffering from PTSD symptoms would be better served in rehabilitation rather than being disciplined for not fighting.[9] Rush's ideas served as the cornerstone for early American efforts to better understand PTSD related symptoms and to guide rehabilitation through national government support.[10]

In 1871, Dr. Jacob de Costa published a report of recorded panic attacks in American Civil War soldiers from 1861-1865, and he coined the term "Irritable Heart of the Soldier" to describe instances of cardiac arrhythmia.[11] During the same time period, Dr. Silas Weir Mitchell,

---

[6] Harry M. Ward, *George Washington's Enforcers: Policing the Continental Army* (Carbondale, IL: Southern Illinois University Press, 2006), iiv.

[7] Nidiffer and Leach, 16.

[8] Ward, xi.

[9] Ibid.

[10] Nidiffer and Leach, 21.

[11] Nancy H. Kobrin and Jerry L. Kobrin, "J.M. da Costa M.D. – An American Civil War Converso Physician," *Shofar* 18 (1999): 16.

a neurologist from Jefferson Medical College, studied post-war nerve injuries caused by gunshot wounds, exhaustion, and amputation.[12] Mitchell developed the diagnosis for anxiety problems called *rest cure*. Da Costa and Mitchell collaborated to identify symptoms and propose treatments such as massage, posture correction, and exercise. According to Nancy Kobrin and Jerry Kobrin, this was a first for "American medicine in that it grounded fear of war in physical symptoms, but more important, it elaborated the interrelationship between emotional trauma of the battlefield and the heart through physiology and cardiology."[13] Lack of knowledge on combat mental issues and the nature of military the late nineteenth century added to the problem of PTSD symptoms in the Army.[14]

Unfortunately, two centuries of advances in psychiatry, psychology, and leadership have not altered the fundamental dynamic of human response to stressful experiences in combat. PTSD has been referred to by Army personnel as "one of the signature injuries of the active duty service men and women who are deployed to Afghanistan or Iraq."[15] A 2008 Tactical Commander PTSD Survey reported that 85% of senior military officers who had experienced combat commands rated themselves as technically solid, but felt "neither adequately trained nor educated to apply tactical measures on the battlefield to prevent or mitigate PTSD."[16] The negative impact of PTSD-diagnosed soldiers assigned to units training for war has become a major concern and a critical problem for the Army.

In order for Army leaders to balance the demands and requirements of a unit with the mental health needs of soldiers, leaders must have access to resources. These resources are

---

[12] Ibid., 20.

[13] Ibid., 19.

[14] Ward, xiii.

[15] Brian P. Marx, "Post Traumatic Stress Disorder and Operations Enduring Freedom and Iraqi Freedom: Progress in the Time of Controversy," *Clinical Psychology Review* 29 (2009): 671.

[16] Haycock, 5.

captured and maintained in what the Army calls doctrine. Doctrine has long served as a source from which leaders can acquire professional guidance. Unfortunately, current leadership doctrine remains strangely silent when it comes to the topic of PTSD.

To address the issues of leadership and PTSD, the Army stands to benefit from exploring how to use doctrine as a mechanism to equip its leaders to fight PTSD within its ranks. How might U.S. Army leadership doctrine be modified by transformational leadership theories to assist leaders with challenges such as PTSD? A detailed discussion of modern leadership theories, doctrine, and three historical case studies will serve as the framework for the study of this question.

The research question will be answered by a comprehensive review of the most current leadership literature. The Army's Be, Know, Do (BKD) leadership model, presented in *FM 6-22 Army Leadership*, has some gaps in its application. But, elements of three additional theories – transformational, leader-member exchange (LMX), and situational leadership – augment the BKD leadership model to best assist leaders with issues related to PTSD. To test this hypothesis, this monograph develops an understanding of recent leadership theories to assist in the analysis of the Army-accepted BKD leadership model. Transformational, LMX, and situational leadership theories are highlighted in the literature review in order to provide a perspective on recent leadership developments and to guide leaders who deal with soldiers diagnosed with PTSD.

The review of the BKD leadership model and the three leadership theories determined three criteria. These criteria address multi-leader collaboration towards PTSD, the relationship between the leader and follower with PTSD, and practice of the BKD leadership model initiating social change within an organization comprised of PTSD-diagnosed members. The criteria are applied to historical case studies, providing analysis that reveals gaps on the Army's BKD leadership model. These gaps are addressed by concepts from transformational, LMX, and situational leadership theories, each of which can be used to augment the leadership model.

Several assumptions exist within the construction of the monograph. First, it is assumed that the leaders are an effective agent to combat the effects of PTSD within a unit. Second, it is assumed that this study is applicable on an educational and institutional level. And third, that data from this proposed study may provide Army officers a working framework that could assist leaders in designing the most effective doctrine.

There are several limitations in this monograph that need to be noted. First, the monograph is an analysis of current leadership doctrine, specifically *Field Manual 6-22, Army Leadership,* dated October 2006. Second, although it is acknowledged that programs exist that assist leaders with the effects of PTSD within the Army organization, they are not within the scope of this monograph. It is also acknowledged that numerous leadership theories and styles exist; however, three were selected because of their unique contribution to the research question. Finally, this monograph is not about the medical aspects of PTSD (neurological, biological, and psychological), the effects of PTSD on the family, or the private treatment plans an individual may receive from medical personnel; however, it does acknowledge the importance and relevance of these topics in the treatment of PTSD.

A variety of literature has been written on PTSD, leadership, and the effects of PTSD on the battlefield. An overview of such material is needed to gain understanding of the topic, identify gaps, and develop solutions for the problem. As mentioned, the effects of PTSD on military leadership are the topic of this monograph, and the works of Gary Yukl, Bernard Bass, Ronald Riggio, and Peter Northouse can provide information towards the subject matter.

Literature Review

Despite the fact that "there is no universally agreed on definition of leadership," theories on the traits of a successful leader have been under examination since the early 1800s.[17] Daniel Van Seter and Richard Fields outlined nine eras of leadership development: personality, influences, behavior, situational, contingency, transactional, anti-leadership, culture, and transformational.[18] Within each era, periods of study exist which are further broken down into specific theories.

For the purposes of this monograph, the literature review focuses on the latest era of leadership theory – transformational leadership – which contains the three specific theories analyzed in this monograph. The transformational era represents the latest in the evolutionary development of leadership theory.[19] In this era leadership is characterized by motivation, charisma, internal and external motivators and feedback, and the environment. Theories of this era – to include transformational, LMX, situational and Theory U – focus on inspiration and change as the springboard for improving an individual and an organization.

For over twenty years, the United States Army has used the Be, Know, Do leadership model to describe what Army leadership is and does.[20] The BKD leadership model is presented on the first pages of *Field Manual 6-22, Army Leadership* and serves as the foundation for the basic leadership understanding in the Army. According to the Army, leadership is "the process of influencing people by providing purpose, direction, and motivation while operating to accomplish

---

[17] Mustafa Rejai and Key Phillips, *Leaders and Leadership: An Appraisal of Theory and Research* (Westport, CT: Praeger, 1997), 87.

[18] Eriaan Oelofse, "Core and Peripheral Cultural Values and Their Relationship to Transformational Leadership Attributes of South African Managers," (doctorate thesis, University of Pretoria, 2006): 64.

[19] Gary Yukl, *Leadership in Organizations* (Upper Saddle River, NJ: Prentice Hall, 2002), 433.

[20] U.S. Department of the Army, *Field Manual 6-22, Army Leadership* (Washington, DC: Government Printing Office, 2006), 1-1.

the mission and improving the organization."[21] The BKD leadership model addresses the personal values, competence, and actions of a leader that influence others to achieve successful mission accomplishment.[22]

Leadership elements of the transformational era are streamlined throughout the BKD leadership model.[23] The first element of the BKD leadership model theory, *Be*, stresses the aspect of the leader's character. The Department of Defense defines character as "the courage to do what is right regardless of the circumstance or the consequences."[24] Character is instilled and refined by Army values. These values guide daily actions and provide the framework in which the leader makes decisions. The element of character consists of three components: mental, physical, and emotional.[25] The BKD leadership model acknowledges that some attributes are innate but assumes that many character-building elements can be learned or changed. The mental component describes the inner drive needed to accomplish a task, the self-discipline to master the practice of consistently doing the right thing, the initiative to act without clear instructions, and the judgment to make sound, educated, and ethical decisions. The physical component stresses the importance of health fitness, physical fitness, and professional bearing. The emotional component details the importance of self-control, balance, and both personal and professional. However, the *Be* component of the Army character does not make explicit the application of the leader's individual mental, physical, and emotional characteristics into a hierarchal organization. However, transformational leadership lends itself to capitalizing on the leader's individual

---

[21] Ibid., 1-2.

[22] Ibid., 1-1.

[23] David Campbell and James Dardis, "The 'Be, Know, Do' Model," *HR, Human Resource Planning* (2004), 27.

[24] FM 6-22, 1-4.

[25] Ibid., 1-6.

characteristics, embedding them into the organization through peer teamwork, shared visions, and a positive work environment.

Transformational leadership theory is grounded in three concepts. First, the leader is not a sole provider of leadership; second, the leader empowers followers through example; and third, the leader must collaborate with superiors, peers, and subordinates to envision a path for the organization. Transformational leaders work to transform their subordinates by challenging them to rise above their immediate needs and self-interests.[26] James Burns and Bernard Bass developed this theory to broaden and elevate the interests of employees, generate awareness and acceptance of the purposes and missions of the organization, and stir the employees to look beyond their own self-interests for the good of the overall entity.[27] This theory is based on the ability of a leader to provide vision and empower followers to immerse themselves in that vision until it becomes their own. One of the characteristics frequently used to describe transformational leaders is visionary. Transformational leaders think ahead to where the organization should be and what the organization should look like.[28]

Once organizational vision is created, transformational leaders outline the plan that moves the organization toward that vision. The transformational leadership theory develops a person using personal and professional growth opportunities, and is unconfined by a hierarchal organizational structure. Leaders empower their subordinates through mentally challenging activities, and then place those empowered individuals in a group setting. When a mentally and situationally aware group is formed, the transformational leader provides a direction for the organization, and steps back to see the subordinates work out the task at hand. Communication is

---

[26] Bernard Bass and Ronald Riggio, *Transformational Leadership,* 2nd ed. (Portland, OR: Taylor and Francis, Inc., 2005), 7.

[27] Ibid.,14.

[28] Peter Northouse, *Leadership: Theory and Practice,* 4th ed. (Thousand Oaks, CA: Sage, 2007), 71.

vital to this process – all levels of the organization need to be aware of what is happening and where the organization is headed. The transformational leader remains committed and involved to see more long-term, definitive goals met. The intent of the transformational leader is to develop a new system for the organization and incorporate that system into the organization dynamic. According to Thomas Mannarelli, "Transformational leaders distinguish themselves by offering an exciting vision or strategy that followers internalize so that successfully enacting their leader's vision becomes not just a job, but also a path towards self-fulfillment."[29] Transformational leadership concepts flourish in an organization that is flattened by leadership style, has an experienced populace, and is faced with crisis, instability, mediocrity, or disenchantment.[30]

The *Know* element of BKD leadership focuses on what the leader must know in order to be competent as an effective leader, and describes the need for leaders to develop both themselves and their subordinates. The *Know* element requires leaders to understand problem solving, tactics, resources management, accountability, and systems in order to shape a leader's identity and reinforce the leader's decisions.[31] Conceptual skills allow leaders to understand ideas, creatively think, and critically reason from experience. However, the *Know* component does not make explicit the importance of the leader and follower relationship, or how to integrate the organic knowledge and talent in the team with action that moves the organization forward.

However, LMX leadership theory attempts to explain the quality of each dyadic relationship of the leader and follower and its effects on the organizational outcomes overtime.[32] The LMX leadership theory focuses on the linkages that leaders experience with each

---

[29] Thomas Mannarelli, "Accounting for Leadership" Charismatic, Transformational Leaders through Reflection and Self-Awareness," *Accountancy Ireland* 38 (2006), 46.

[30] Bass and Riggio, 19.

[31] FM 6-22, 1-1.

[32] Yukl, 131.

subordinate. The relationships can range from a mutual trusting and respectful relationship to a

leader follower relationship characterized by orders.[33] Positive relationships between leaders and

followers entail input, information, issues, recommendations, and solutions collectively

developed by all members of the organization. A negative relationship between leaders and

followers is characterized by a leader's traditional supervisory approach, to which the follower

responds by helping the leader based on outlined assigned responsibilities. If implemented

appropriately, this leadership theory can be very effective because it uses the entire capability of

all of its members to solve problems that challenge the organization.[34]

The *Do* element of the BKD model describes the normal actions taken by a leader.[35] The

Do element is comprised of three components: influencing, operating, and improving.[36] This

element emphasizes the need for leaders to develop "interpersonal, conceptual, and technical

skills that allow them to influence others."[37] Interpersonal skills empower leaders to coach, teach,

and mentor subordinates while increasing proficiency in communication of intent. Leaders

influence personnel by making decisions for the betterment of the organization, communicating,

and motivating personnel to execute decisions.[38] The *Do* component stresses the critical aspect of

improving the organizational capacity to conduct tasks, promote personal development, and foster

an environment for self-improvement.[39] The *Do* component does not make explicit the need of a

---

[33] Northouse, 77.

[34] Robert Lussier and Christopher Achua, *Leadership: Theory, Application, and Skill Development* (Mason, OH: Southwestern, 2009), 238.

[35] FM 6-22, 1-2.

[36] Ibid.

[37] Campbell and Dardis, 28.

[38] Yukl, 12.

[39] Campbell and Dardis, 33.

leader to understand the environment to an extent that allows social change to improve the organization.

Leaders who understand the operating environment can "create a solid framework upon which to build a picture of the conditions that will shape" the decisions a leader must make.[40] Situational leadership theory suggests that effective leadership takes place through the process of providing solutions to critical problems the leader faces, which could involve instituting social change in the organization.[41] Two fundamental concepts within the situational leadership theory are the leadership style and the maturity level of the individual or organization. Leadership styles are characterized by the task-relationship behavior of both the leader and the follower, which are called leadership behaviors. These four behaviors are telling behavior (S1), selling behavior (S2), participating behavior (S3), and delegating behavior (S4). The theory suggests that effective leaders will adapt according to the situation, and can use all forms of leadership style behavior.[42] In correlation to the leadership style, the follower's maturity level is categorized by behavior and determines which of the four types of leadership style to use. The first level of maturity (M1) represents the level at which the follower is unwilling or unable to take on responsibility. The M2 level measures the maturity level of the follower who is unable to take on responsibility, but willing to work at the task. A higher measure, M3, describes a follower who can complete tasks, but lacks confidence. Finally, the M4 level is the maturity level in which a follower takes on tasks confidently, and assumes responsibility for the tasks.[43] Situational leaders collectively use the two

---

[40] U.S. Department of the Army, *Field Manual 3-0, Operations* (Washington, DC: Government Printing Office, February, 2008), 1-3.

[41] Oelofse, 71.

[42] Paul Hersey and Kenneth Blanchard, *Management of Organizational Behavior: Utilizing Human Resources*, 4th ed. (Englewood Cliffs, NJ: Prentice Hall, 1982), 152.

[43] Oelofse, 71.

concepts to make the best decisions in the environment in which they are operating and base these decisions on the need to create change within the organization.

A related concept from situational leadership theory is Theory U. This concept offers the idea that a leader offers subordinates new ways of looking at old problems and emphasizes teaching his or her followers to search for sensible solutions to challenging problems.[44] This approach increases the leader's appeal because it places value in the confidence and self-worth of followers. According to Theory U, leaders exert tremendous influence on followers, which is important for transformational leaders. In situational leadership, the importance of leaders is characterized by providing vision and a sense of mission, instilling pride in and among the group members, and gaining the respect and trust of members in the organization.

The BKD leadership model and the three leadership theories discussed attempt to enhance the effectiveness of a leader within an organization. The BKD model of leadership outlines leader's personal character, competence, and daily actions as attributes displayed by a leader towards organizational members. Transformational leadership expands the BKD attributes as the theory recognizes that leadership can emerge anywhere in an organization and leader collaboration is paramount to the success of the organization.[45] Leader-member exchange leadership theory expands leadership concepts by focusing on the leader-follower relationship and considers the input, responsibility, solutions, and feedback of all organization members. Situational leadership theory further acknowledges the environment in which the leader is operating. A leader's understanding of an environment impacts the choice of leadership style within the organization and how it is applied to change the environment to best benefit the organization.

_____

[44] Hersey and Blanchard, 155.

[45] Campbell and Dardis, 24.

Although the study of leadership is not monolithic, leadership theorists maintain a few consistencies in the research. First, there is a relationship between leaders which identifies the strengths and weaknesses of an organization and establishes the criteria of leadership collaboration. Second, leader and follower involvement can yield positive results for the organization as a whole. Third, the manner in which a leader responds to a leadership challenge affects its outcome, which informs a framework for analyzing social change within an organization. Finding the balance of the relationship, involvement, and response is critical when defining a successful leadership experience.[46]

Leaders in today's Army must balance the needs of the soldier diagnosed with PTSD and military organizational requirements. They understand that PTSD is in its formations and affects the individual, peers, subordinates, and leaders. Any gaps between limited and overt levels of PTSD within an organization can be addressed by encouraging collaboration among leaders, developing trust relationships between leaders and subordinates, and creating social change.

Methodology

Army doctrine provides military forces with a common understanding and lexicon of how to conduct operations. Doctrine is extremely important to soldiers because it explains how the Army, as an institution, organizes, trains, and equips soldiers to face global challenges. For leaders, the BKD leadership model has served as the lexicon for over twenty years.[47] Ongoing operations demonstrated shortcomings in current doctrine, which are clarified using recent leadership theories and historical experience. Within the Army, while in prolonged conflicts, the challenge of PTSD requires the attention of leaders.[48] Leadership development programs

---

[46] Hersey and Blanchard, 157.

[47] U.S. Department of the Army, *Field Manual 22-100, Military Leadership* (Washington, DC: Government Printing Office, October, 1983), 1-3.

[48] Haycock, 8.

13

applicable to the challenges the Army faces are necessary to posture organizational success.[49]

"Leadership in today's operational environment is often the difference between success and failure."[50] Army *Field Manual 3-0, Operations* details that the role of leadership is central to all Army operations and influences people by providing purpose, direction, and motivation, while operating to accomplish the mission and improving the organization. Leadership and the warrior ethos sustain soldiers during the brutal realities of combat and help them cope with the ambiguities of complex military operations. Leaders create conditions for success – organizing, equipping, training, and leading soldiers to accomplish operational missions are the goals of leaders.[51]

The selected case studies are taken from World War I, World War II, and Vietnam experience. Each historical example outlines a period during which American military leadership encountered PTSD, or one of its predecessors, on a large scale. The first case study describes the American reaction to shell shock during World War I. The second case study presents American servicemen and the combat stress of World War II. The third case study describes the American military experience with PTSD in Vietnam.

Using an understanding of the BKD leadership model, together with the transformational, leader-member, and situational leadership theories, three concepts emerge that serve as the criterion for the examination of experience drawn from military history. These criteria serve as the driver of this inquiry of the BKD leadership model and the framework in which the specific criteria were developed. The criteria address multi-leader collaboration towards PTSD, the

---

[49] Yulk, 15.

[50] FM 3-0, 4-2.

[51] Ibid., 1-1.

relationship between the leader and follower with PTSD, and practice of leading social change within an organization comprised of PTSD diagnosed members.

As presented in the literature review, leadership requires a relationship between leaders themselves, and military leadership is no different. It is from this concept that the first criterion was developed: Is there evidence of leaders collaborating to address PTSD? Using this criterion as a springboard, the monograph investigates leadership collaboration on the problem of PTSD. Evident, non-evident, or ambiguous evidence of a relationship between leaders will serve as the evidentiary scale.

Second, leadership requires a leader and follower relationship. A military leader and follower relationship enables hierarchal organization in which leaders order followers into a wide range of environments. It is from this concept that the second criterion was developed: Is there evidence of practices that developed relationships between leader and follower? From the perspective of this criterion, the leader-follower relationship is investigated to gain understanding of the relationships of leaders and followers. Evident, non-evident, or ambiguous evidence of a relationship between leaders and followers will serve as the evidentiary scale.

Third, the concept of social change is a leader's legacy to an organization. The concept of social change is the slowest to initiate, develop, and implement. Military organizations have a social culture that was derived from various experiences such as war and the men and women who fought in those conflicts. This concept provides the third criterion: evidence of practices in the Army that led to social change regarding PTSD. From this criterion, evidence of social change is investigated to gain understanding of PTSD within an organization and social changes that emerged due to PTSD in the formation. Evident, non-evident, or ambiguous evidence of social change within an organization will serve as the evidentiary scale. After the evaluation of the criteria and data collection is complete for each case study, a table of evidence is established, and an assessment to apply transformational, LMX, and situational leadership theory literature is developed. At the conclusion of the case study, a table of all the evidentiary scale is presented.

Analysis

War Neurosis in World War I

World War I (1914-1918) began as a war of movement and maneuver, during which nominal psychological reactions were observed.[52] As movement became restricted, trench warfare became the forefront of conflict. Following the transition from movement and maneuver tactics to trench warfare, British soldiers presented signs of depression, anxiety, nervousness, and paralysis.[53] Initially, the British physicians did not treat the emerging symptoms as a mental disorder because at the time it was believed that only women had psychological disorders. So, naturally, the physicians turned to actions on the battlefield for answers to the problems of their soldiers.[54] In 1915, British physicians described neurological system injuries as "shell shock," the cause of which was believed to be a change in atmospheric pressure caused by an exploding shell near a soldier. This pressure resulted in harm to the nervous system similar to that of a concussion. However, it was soon realized that most cases did not involve exploding ordnance and the diagnostic term was changed to "war neurosis."[55] By 1916, more than 40% of the British casualties in combat were diagnosed as causalities of war neurosis.[56]

---

[52] Todd C Helmus and Russell W. Glenn, "Steeling the Mind: Combat Stress Reactions and Their Implications for Urban Warfare" (Monograph, The Rand Corporation, 2005), 10.

[53] Franklin D. Jones, "Traditional Warfare Combat Stress Casualties," *War Psychiatry* (1995): 35-61.

[54] Ben Shephard, "Shell-Shock on the Somme," *RUSI Journal* (June 1996): 51-56.

[55] Anthony Babington, *Shell Shock: A History of the Changing Attitudes to War Neurosis* (London: Leo Cooper, 1997), 3. According to this source, the term Not Yet Diagnosed Nervous (N.Y.D.N) was applied to soldiers experiencing unexplained neurological symptoms.

[56] D.H. Marlow, "Delayed and Immediate Onset Post Traumatic Stress Disorder," *Social Psychiatry and Psychiatric Epidemiology* (1991): 3.

Societal norms exerted a masculine perspective, which discouraged the reporting of mental health problems in men. Some commanders, medical personnel, and soldiers believed that the outward expression of mental health symptoms was a sign of weakness.[57] Lieutenant-General Sir Aymer Hunter-Weston said, "Cowards constituted a danger to the war effort, and the sanction of the death penalty was designed to frighten men more than the prospects of facing the enemy."[58] Men who presented symptoms of war neurosis were often disciplined through military justice, and, in some cases, sentenced to death.[59] As the war continued and the number of cases of war neurosis rose, treatment plans began to evolve. If a soldier was diagnosed with war neurosis, that soldier was referred to the medical staff and pulled further from the front lines. In some cases, soldiers were sent to Great Britain and admitted to psychiatric wards. However, even with an increase of evacuation from the front lines, 60%-70% of the cases seen in Great Britain were treated in less than a week and returned into theater to continue fighting.[60]

In 1917, the United States prepared for war and, using British experience, determined treatment methods for war neurosis. To learn about war neurosis, the Army deployed Dr. Thomas Salmon, who was assigned lead psychiatrists for a neuropsychiatric service plan for the Army. After observing the French and British centers, Dr. Salmon returned home and suggested that the treatment of war neurosis be treated as close to the battle lines as possible.[61] After treatment, the soldier could return to the unit and return to duty. Dr. Salmon's method of treatment was outlined as "proximity, immediacy, and expectancy."[62]

---

[57] Helmus and Glenn, 11.

[58] Martin Gilbert, *The First World War: A Complete History* (New York: Henry Holt, 1994), 275.

[59] Shephard, 53.

[60] Marlow, 4.

[61] Helmus and Glenn,12.

[62] Kenneth L. Artiss, "Human Behavior Under Stress: From Combat to Social Psychiatry," *Military Medicine* 28 (1963): 1011-1015.

Even with advanced planning to address war neurosis, American leaders, especially

General John Pershing, were shocked at the number of war neurosis cases. During the Argonne

offensive, estimates range from 35-45% of soldiers experienced war neurosis symptoms, which

caused an evacuation from theater.[63] The Meuse-Argonne Offensive was the largest U.S.

engagement of the war, beginning on September 26, 1918 and ending November 11, 1918. In the

three weeks of battle, the total number of American dead numbered 18,000.[64] Sergeant Gordon

Fisher, who was present in the Meuse-Argonne Offensive, explained:

> I went further along and looked into the next dug-out and there was a guardsman in there.
> They talk about the psychology of fear. He was a perfect example. I can see that
> Guardsman now! His face was yellow, he was shaking all over, and I said to him, "What
> the hell are you doing here?" He said, "I can't go. I can't do it. I daren't go!" Now, I was
> pretty ruthless in those days and I said to him, "Look, I'm going up the line and when I
> come back if you're still here I'll shoot you!" . . . when I came back, thank God, he'd
> gone. He'd got genuine shell shock. We didn't realize that at the time. We used to think it
> was cowardice, but we learned later on that there was such a thing as shell shock. Poor
> chap, he couldn't help it. It could happen to anybody. [65]

By the end of the offensive, more than 80,000 cases were treated by British and

American medical staffs.[66] After the offensive, General Pershing visited the wounded in French

and American field hospitals and treatment tents. His visits brightened the seemingly dismal

environment of the hospital as he walked through rows and rows of men injured as a result of his

orders. General Pershing was humbled by the men and often prayed that God would be with

them.[67]

---

[63] Edgar Jones, Nicola Fear, and Simon Wesley, "Shell Shock and Mild Traumatic Brain Injury: A Historical Review," *AM Psychiatry* 164, no.11 (November 2007), 1641.

[64] Ibid.

[65] Lyn Macdonald, *1915, The Death of Innocence* (New York: Henry Holt and Company, 1995), 476.

[66] John Simkin, "The Medical Treatment of Shell Shock," through http://www.spartacus.schoolnet.co.uk/ (accessed June 1, 2010).

[67] Donald Smythe, *Pershing: Generals of the Armies* (Bloomington, IN: Indiana University Press, 1986), 156.

American military efforts in World War I projected the United States as a global military power. Soldiers returned home as heroes and citizen pride was unwavering. War neurosis came home with soldiers as well, and treatment was conducted by civilian hospitals. Subsequent study of World War I included an examination of war neurosis and its effect on the soldier and battle. As the United States military readjusted back to garrison, the education of mental health continued and assisted leaders to prepare for future battles.[68]

Criteria Analysis of War Neurosis

As battle lines stabilized in World War I, trench warfare on the battlefield ensued and brought psychiatric problems of soldiers to the forefront. Immediately following the entrance into the war, military leaders observed the effects of war neurosis in British formations and made attempts to provide psychiatric assistance as forward as possible. Military leaders lacked a complete understanding of war neurosis' causes and effects but, one thing was certain: combat power was affected by war neurosis, and it seemed to be linked to the frequency of combat. As the frequency of combat increased, so did the frequency of war neurosis patients.[69]

Evidence of leaders collaborating in address war neurosis existed because actions were taken by military leaders and medical personnel to treat soldiers with war neurosis even without a complete understanding of the best treatment method. The World War I historical experience reveals American leaders observed the war neurosis dilemma of the British and attempted to treat this emerging problem as American forces entered the war. General Pershing personally visited many field hospitals full of soldiers with injuries. "Pershing himself was understandably fatigued and depressed. Once leaving a hospital Pershing moaned to his driver, 'I feel like I have the

---

[68] Helmus and Glenn, 12.

[69] Jones, Fear, and Wesley, 1641.

19

weight of the world on my shoulders'. He sobbed and cried out to his dead wife that he could not go on."[70]

As the symptoms of war neurosis emerged, medical providers sought to assist the soldier. Four concepts developed during the American Expeditionary Forces (AEF) combat experience in World War I. First, the precedent was set for the need for military psychiatric services for all men in units.[71] As the war continued, a shift in focus from a reaction to shell bombardment to an emotional disorder prevailed. Second, treatment was temporary in nature. The goal of medical staffs was to return the soldier to the line as fast as possible. Ronald Shaffer suggested that the main goal for AEF leaders and medical personnel was to win the war, even if it meant a "quick fix" for war neurosis exposed soldiers.[72] Third, vague explanations of symptoms by soldiers hindered treatment methods. Additionally, the inconsistent treatment methods of medical providers failed to collectively gain evidence to support the best classifications of treatments to solve the problem.

Evidence from the historical experience reveals an ambiguous relationship between leaders and followers addressing war neurosis. This was largely due to the lack of knowledge on the subject matter and varying treatment methods based on rank. Leaders learned on the battlefield about the effects war neurosis had on troop strength, morale, and mission effectiveness. Officers were less likely to break down in combat operational than enlisted personnel, but were more likely to break down over an extended period of persistent combat. An enlisted man's treatment was shorter in duration and almost always returned to the trenches,

---

[70] Smythe, 208.

[71] Barbara Jones, "Post-traumatic Stress Disorder in the United States Legal Culture: An Historical Perspective from World War I through the Vietnam Conflict" (doctoral thesis, University of Minnesota, 1995), 33.

[72] Ronald Shaffer, "The Treatment of 'Shell Shock' Cases in the AEF: A Microcosm of the War Welfare State" in *America in the Great War: The Rise of the War Welfare State* (New York: Oxford University Press, 1991): 199-212.

whereas officers' treatment was more extensive. War neurosis affected officers and enlisted soldiers but different treatment were applied to the groups. Enlisted men witnessed the more comprehensive treatment for officers, contrasted with the short stints of aid given to enlisted soldiers.[73] As a result, a divide between officers and enlisted emerged. Eric Leed posited "in war, as in peace, the notion that disease could be without physiological signs, that could have a purely behavioral expression, seems to be the exclusive property of the higher social orders."[74]

Presence of evidence for social change regarding PTSD in the military exists within historical experience. Because of the emergence of war and the persistence of PTSD, the commander's ability to fight the enemy was affected. As an organization, the Army changed. The American experience in World War I began with a baseline understanding of war neurosis derived from observation of the British military. Dr. Salmon established multi-echelon treatment facilities in which patients were treated as close to the battle line as possible and possibly removed farther away based on the severity of the problem.[75] The projection of the mental health capacity forward increased the ability to seek treatment and the speed of return to the front line.

Recognized by his efforts to treat and return soldiers to the line, Dr. Salmon was appointed as an advisor to General Perishing and continued to investigate the depth and breadth of was neurosis in the formation. General Pershing and medical personnel did not know the complete effects of war neurosis but did know through observation of the British and first-hand knowledge that the emergence of war neurosis hindered military effectiveness. The Army felt these hindrances in decreased personnel strength and morale, indicating a need for leaders to take action that set the conditions for how the Army was going to face this new threat.

---

[73] Jones, 35.

[74] Leed, 164.

[75] Helmus and Glenn, 12.

The historical experience of war neurosis in World War I led to further study of mental health as a result of combat operations. As outlined, war neurosis was a problem that was identified and learned about through the actions on the battlefield. Henry Mintzberg suggested sometimes the environment simply changed in ways that were not predictable and informed leaders recognized the limitations of the initial strategies early enough to face the new environment and make changes.[76] Dr. Salmon and military leader efforts attempted to address war neurosis with the information gathered and the use of medicine in the formation.

However, the divide of treatment methods hindered the formation. Officers seemed to be cared for more extensively, while enlisted men were sent forward as soon as possible. Selected treatment programs based on rank, race, or other ambiguous factors sent soldiers back to the trenches unwell and feeling undervalued.[77] Evidence of leadership collaboration, leaders and followers addressing PTSD, and evidence of social change in the historical experience resulted in the following assessment:

	Criteria 1: Leader Collaboration	Criteria 2: Leader/Follower Relationship	Criteria 3: Social Change in the Army
World War I	E	A	E

Figure 1. Summary Chart of Historical Experience #1

Figure 1 presents an evident (E), non-evident (NE), or ambiguous (A) summary chart of Case Study #1 to provide evidence to support the evaluation criteria. Evident (E) is favorable, ambiguous (A) represents null evidence, and non-evident (NE) is no evidence to support the criterion.

---

[76] Henry Mintzberg, *The Rise and Fall of Strategic Planning* (New York: The Free Press, 1994), 285.

[77] Eric Leed, *No Man's Land: Combat and Identity in World War I* (Cambridge, UK: Cambridge University Press, 1981), 164.

As war neurosis materialized in the formation, leaders adapted by sending medical treatment forward and attempted to change the previous negative stigma associated with men and mental illness through the leader's action towards the problem. The World War I historical experience highlights leadership capability to adapt towards an unknown problem, to set the conditions for success within the formation simply by understanding the environment and to use courage to inflict change.

In the historical experience, the BKD model of leadership is evidence of leaders collaborating and creating social change with regard to war neurosis in the military. One area of concern is the relationship between leaders and followers, which has been a foundation for the BKD leadership model. The *Do* element is directly related to influence because without influence the leader cannot continue to have impact.

Combat Fatigue in World War II

As the United States entered World War II, military leaders were determined to reduce psychiatric losses of the scale suffered in the previous World War.[78] The United States military organized for war, believing that soldier selection and screening served as the solution to mental health problems.[79] Harry Sullivan, a chief psychologist in the Selective Service System of the Veterans Administration viewed the concept of screening as a two-fold success. First, the system satisfied the wartime problem of preventing unfit soldiers in combat. Second, the system circumvented strain the economic cost of long- term treatment for mass combat stress patients as it did in WWI.[80]

---

[78] Shephard, 54.

[79] Marlow, 6.

[80] Harry S. Sullivan, "Psychiatry and the National Defense," in Harry S. Sullivan, *The Fusion of Psychiatry and Social Science* (New York: Norton, 1964): 2.

23

The idea of screening before and during service was appealing but views soon changed. Potential service members were rejected for claims of prior anxiety disorders, educational shortcomings, or neurotic personalities.[81] Screening systems were tested in the early phases of World War II. Early combat experience called into question the efficacy of screening systems. United States Marines at the Battle of Guadalcanal from August through November 1942 endured poor living conditions, food, and unending contact from the enemy.[82] As a result, war neurosis cases were high and hospitals were once again overrun with mental health problems of the combat veteran. In 1943, during the North African Campaign, "one of the first times American troops faced the German Army, rates of battle fatigue were so high at times that replacements could not come fast enough."[83] During the Battle of Kasserine, a poorly trained American division clashed with Rommel's forces. One American soldier noted "a feeling of helplessness as he watched shells from his unit's short-barreled low-velocity 75mm Howitzers bounce off the attacking German Panzers."[84] Men were demoralized and mentally distraught as they faced the reality that their force was ill-equipped for the engagements in Africa. The clinical picture mirrored the effects of shell shock and war neurosis the Allies experienced a few decades earlier in World War I.

General Omar Bradley grew especially concerned and requested assistance from civilian experts. Dr. Frederick Hanson and Dr. Louis Tureen volunteered and deployed overseas, and they reignited the principle of the need for forward-based medical treatment facilities throughout the Allied operating lines. At various treatment facilities, Hanson and Tureen reportedly returned

---

[81] A. J. Glass, "Lessons Learned," in A.J. Glass and R.J. Bernucci, eds. *The History of Neuropsychiatry in World War II,* Vol. 1, *Zone of Interior* (Washington, DC: Government Printing Office, 1966): 735-760.

[82] Shephard, 223.

[83] Nidiffer and Leach, 9.

[84] Marlow, 6.

30% of patients back to their respective units within thirty hours and 70% of patients within seventy-two hours of arrival to the facility.[85] The team of doctors suggested to General Bradley that the name 'war neurosis' be changed to 'combat exhaustion' in order to allude to the breakdown as a more natural, short-term problem. Some progress of combat exhaustion treatment existed, but efforts were not in full measure towards the end of 1943.

The well-publicized slapping of a combat exhaustion patient by General George Patton fueled a public uproar and propelled the issue of combat exhaustion to the forefront of society. In response, the War Department authorized a psychiatrist for the division's Table of Organization and Equipment (TOE).[86] The use of Dr. Salmon's idea of forward psychiatry and the efforts of Dr. Hanson and Dr. Tureen were necessary, given the high rates of combat exhaustion that existed throughout the war.[87]

An analysis of Allied medical reports indicated one of four patients were admitted for mental health problems, and one out of three American soldiers serving in Europe during World War II received a diagnosis of combat exhaustion.[88] Glass posited that 400,000 U.S. service members were sent home for psychological problems, a number roughly the equivalent to the total number killed and missing in World War II combat operations.[89]

American military efforts in World War II contributed immensely to the end of Nazi Germany and Japan. A generation of heroes returned home and was given a very progressive

---

[85] C.S. Drayer and A.J. Glass, "Introduction," in A.J. Glass, ed., *Medical Department, United States Army, Neuropsychiatry in World War II,* Vol. 2, *Overseas Theaters* (Washington DC: Office of the Surgeon General, 1973), ii.

[86] Helmus and Glenn, 15.

[87] Ibid.

[88] Ginzberg, 124.

[89] Glass, 997.

veterans package, the GI Bill of Rights.[90] The United States government provided military

members with education, training, employment, and housing assistance. "Never has a nation

lavished so many material benefits upon its heroes. From subsidized education to privileged

ocean travel for their war brides, World War II veterans received a rich bounty."[91] With a nation

victorious over the Nazis and abundance of support for the veterans, it was a surprise when

combat fatigue did not dissolve after all the home front rehabilitation programs ended. Even with

the positive impact of soldiers returning home to benefits and opportunities, fewer than half felt

their contributions were appreciated and many felt alienated from the communities.[92] The

problem of combat exhaustion of World War II veterans remained a predominant diagnosis in

veteran's hospitals while research of the problem continued.

Criteria Analysis of Combat Exhaustion

Leaders collaborating to address combat exhaustion was evident throughout the historical

experience of World War II. U.S. military preparations for combat included mental health

considerations for its soldiers. Initially, the United States government did not want to be tied to

exhaustive medical bills and compensations as it was in World War I. In an attempt to alleviate

mental health issues in its military formations and the high cost of treatment, the government

conducted rigorous screening to all of its potential service members. Overall, 1.6 million men

were denied military service due to potential psychological shortfalls.[93]

---

[90] Jones, 56.

[91] Davis Ross, *Preparing for Ulysses: Politics and Veterans During World War II* (New York: Columbia University Press, 1969), 3.

[92] Jones, 60.

[93] Glass, 735-737.

As combat operations began, American commanders were shocked that the screening did not solve the problems of combat exhaustion in its formation. Just as in World War I, military leadership was reactive to combat exhaustion as combat operations continued to increase in lethality. Herbert X. Spiegel, a psychiatrist who worked with Dr. Hanson and Dr. Tureen, offered:

> It seemed to me that the drive was more a positive than a negative one. It was love more than hate. Love manifested by 1) regard for their comrades who shared the same dangers, 2) respect for their platoon leader or company commander who led them wisely and backed them with everything at his command, 3) concern for their reputation with their commander and leaders, and 4) an urge to contribute to the task and success of their group and unit. . They seemed to be fighting for somebody rather than against somebody.[94]

The relationship soldiers had with peers and leaders enabled the soldier to cope with exhaustion and to prevent breakdown and longer-term psychological damage.[95]

Evidence from the historical experience revealed an ambiguous relationship between leaders and followers when addressing PTSD. In some units, the relationship between leader and subordinated was positive and their units demonstrated low combat exhaustion cases. The 442nd Regimental Combat Team, out of Hawaii, experienced low rates of combat stress cases throughout the Italian and German campaigns. This unit was the most decorated unit in the Army to date, and had within its ranks twenty-one Medal of Honor recipients. The men thought in some of the toughest battles of World War II and were well respected. Teamwork of members was unmatched and every soldier played an important role in the units' success.

"Everyone in the Army is part of a team, and all members have an inherent responsibly to that team."[96] Soldiers who embraced learning about combat stress and its symptoms, and leaders who addressed mental health as being just as important as physical health were far less likely to

---

[94] Herbert Spiegel, "Preventive Psychiatry with Combat Troops," *American Journal of Psychiatry* 101 (November 1944): 311-312.

[95] Marlow, 5.

[96] FM 6-22, viii.

"allow" combat stress symptoms in their units. In some Airborne and Ranger units, rates of combat stress were dramatically lower than those of regular infantry units because the leadership culture concerning combat stress was a top-down, down-up collective approach to educate soldiers and leaders on mental health advancements that treated issues both individually and as a team.[97]

However, not all organizations were equal in their success against combat exhaustion. The 169th Infantry Regiment operating in the Pacific Theater was characterized by low morale and incompetent leadership.[98] In the unit's first engagement, 10% of their personnel losses were due to combat exhaustion. As the regiment continued to fight, leadership problems, soldier discipline issues, and combat exhaustion rates soared reaching an estimate of over 50% by late 1942.[99]

The historical experience reveals evidence of social change regarding combat exhaustion and the Army. After scrutinizing screening criteria from a psychiatry perspective, the emergence of combat exhaustion in World War II opened the idea that the stresses of combat were likely to affect a pre-disposed group of people.[100] The development of what causes combat exhaustion shifted from a strictly predisposition of some to the vulnerability of every man. Although stigma may accompany combat exhaustion, no one was exempt from the scrutiny. Mass numbers of

---

[97] Marlow, 5.

[98] Jules V. Coleman, "Division Psychiatry in the Southwest Pacific Area," in W. Mullins and A.J. Glass, eds., *The History of Neuropsychiatry in World War II,* Volume II (Washington, DC: Government Printing Office, 1973): 637.

[99] Coleman, 637.

[100] Jones, 62.

combat stress cases, spanning through race, rank, and level of exposure, led to the belief that all combatants could become causalities of combat exhaustion.[101]

From a military perspective, some lessons learned in World War I were not applied in World War II. The echeloning of forward care outlined by Dr. Salmon in World War I was not implemented until rates of combat exhaustion cases skyrocketed. Leaders, such as General Bradley and commanders in the 442nd Regimental Combat team sought to educate soldiers on the signs of combat exhaustion and promote teamwork within the organization in efforts to prevent the problem.

Evidence of leadership collaboration, leaders and followers addressing PTSD, and evidence of social change in the historical experience resulted in the following assessment:

	Criteria 1: Leader Collaboration	Criteria 2: Leader/Follower Relationship	Criteria 3: Social Change in the Army
World War II	E	A	E

Figure 2. Summary Chart of Historical Experience #2

Figure 2 presents an evident (E), non-evident (NE), or ambiguous (A) summary chart of Case Study #2 to provide evidence to support the evaluation criteria. Evident (E) is favorable, ambiguous (A) represents null evidence, and non-evident (NE) is no evidence to support the criterion.

The Army attempted to remove combat exhaustion within its formation by screening personnel registered for service obligations and unifying formations to face combat exhaustion as a team against an enemy. All efforts were valuable in reducing combat exhaustion but were not enough to remove the problem. The effects of World War II combat exhaustion cases in veteran's

---

[101] Roy L. Swank and Walter E. Marchland, "Combat Neuroses," *Archives of Neurology and Psychiatry* 55 (March 1946): 212.

hospitals were staggering. In 1943, veteran's hospitals still housed over 68,000 World War I veterans, but the facilities received an additional 80,000 World War II veterans with combat exhaustion.[102] In World War I, leaders witnessed the emergence of war neurosis during war. In World War II, leaders applied the wrong solution, which was screening to the root cause of combat exhaustion, which caused leaders to react to combat exhaustion after it took root in the formation. As discussed in the literature review, one of the BKD models of leadership tenets is Know. Leadership requires knowing about the environment, emerging problems, tactics, operating systems, and the human dimension in an organization.

Combat Stress in Vietnam

As the United States entered Vietnam, military leaders focused medical treatment in theater at large bases, and as the war continued, uncoiled forward medical facilities as soldier missions were conducted throughout the entire country. United States participation in the Vietnam War from 1955-1975 has been one of the most debated conflicts of American history.[103] From a national strategic perspective, the approach of the war in some respects unfolded differently than other conflicts. For example, the escalation of conflict was unique. Phillip Davidson posited that the Vietnam War should be characterized into three phases: 1955-1965, characterized by an insurgency and counterinsurgency engagement with a few conventional battles; 1965-1968, a combination of insurgency and conventional war; and 1968-1975, a

---

[102] Jones, 62.

[103] Marlow, 6.

30

conventional fight.[104] "Unlike the Korean War or WWII, Vietnam engagements were short, bloody in which the losing force broke off contact and quit the field."[105]

The Vietnam War once again demonstrated the effects of mental health in military organizations. Prior to the Vietnam War, a cause and effect relationship existed between the frequency and duration of combat and the incidence of combat stress causalities.[106] In a cause and effect model, if combat actions rise, there is an increase of combat stress cases. To best prepare for combat stress cases, the Army developed United States Army Vietnam regulation Number 40-34, which ordered treatment of combat stress cases in theater.[107] Psychiatrists, social workers, surgeons, and psychologists were used at brigade level. Field evacuation hospitals were equipped with teams of mental health providers, nurses, and psychiatric wards.[108] Combat stress cases were thought to be low because for the first time, a trained medical capability was nearly co-located with units, and in the early part of the war units went out on relatively short missions and returned to a relatively safe base of operations.[109]

However, as years of war continued, cases of combat stress began to emerge. The Vietnam War produced an extremely low proportion of combat stress casualties, which appeared emerged during the initial phases of combat operations; however, massive numbers of combat stress casualties during the latter phases and post war years.[110] The greatest increase of combat

_____

[104] Paul Davidson, *Vietnam at War* (New York: Oxford University Press, 1991), 43-51.

[105] Harold G. Moore, and Joseph Galloway, *We Were Soldier Once . . . and Young* (New York: Random House, 1992), 105-135.

[106] Jones, 79.

[107] USARV Regulation Number 40-34, dated March 30, 1966. This regulation placed emphasis on trained psychiatric personnel embedded with and operating within the same battle space as the units conducting operations.

[108] Jones, 82.

[109] Ibid.

[110] Marlow, 7.

stress cases were from 1969-1971 as American forces transitioned into less intense combat operations.[111] Ronald Spector stated "By 1970 there were more than twice as many hospital admissions for psychosis, psychoneurosis, and character and behavior disorders as there had been in 1967. In terms of man-days lost, neuropsychiatric problems had become the second leading disease problem in the theater."[112] Leadership and medical personnel were shocked at what seemed to be the dislocation of high intensity combat and combat stress. A new epidemic was surfacing within the military, and leaders on the battlefield believed combat intensity was not the sole source of the blame.[113]

Military leaders and civilian physiatrists began to investigate what had changed since the inception of the war. [114] Three concepts were identified as possible reasons for the sudden increase of combat stress cases towards the end of the war and for years following. First, the vision of what winning looked like by government leaders changed as the war progressed. Second, the dependency of prescription drugs administered by health professionals and the use illegal narcotics by military members to mask signs of combat stress became common. Third, the guilt soldiers felt afterwards attributed to the upsurge in combat stress.[115]

Military professionals believed that, in the beginning of the war, the possibility of winning existed within units, but as time progressed, the belief vanished.[116] During the Vietnamization period, the "psychological consequences of a war fought where the number

---

[111] Ibid.

[112] Ronald Spector, *After Tet* (New York The Free Press, 1993), 30.

[113] Herbert Hendin and Ann Pollinger Hass, *Wounds of War* (New York: Basic Books, 1984), 18.

[114] Franklin Del Jones, and Arnold W. Johnson, Jr., "Medical and Psychiatric Treatment Policy and Practice in Vietnam," *Journal of Social Issues* 31 (1975): 49-65.

[115] Hendis and Hass, 210-244.

[116] Jones, 83.

killed, rather than terrain gained was the prime objective were enormous."[117] Perceptions of losing by the American people and wavering effort of the American government fueled military member's questions to leadership over tactical decisions, reasons for military presence, and the date for draw down of forces.[118] The political divisiveness surrounding the war, and the lack of support for returning soldiers, contributed to the widespread problems with veterans.[119]

Causes of combat stress were present in the theater of operations as well. Psychologist Norman Camp conducted a study of 135 veteran psychologists who had served in Vietnam to investigate the preponderance of drug use in theater.[120] Camp asserted "Vietnam appears to be the first where drug and alcohol dependency conditions dramatically overshadowed combat reactions."[121] William Datel and Arnold Johnson reported following a survey of 116 Army psychiatrists and general medical officers who served in Vietnam in 1967, "prescribing physicians were of the opinion that prescribed drug treatment was by and large quite influential in reducing the problems presented." [122] During the Tet Offensive and the long withdrawal of soldiers, drug problems rose. By 1969, drug abuse was the main problem, perhaps, the only problem, seen by psychiatrists in theater.[123] As Army leadership became consumed with the increase in drug related incidents, the number of trained psychiatrists decreased.[124] A treatment

---

[117] Hendin and Hass, 233.

[118] Del Jones and Johnson, 52.

[119] Hendis and Hass, 7.

[120] Jones, 84.

[121] Norman M. Camp, *U.S. Army Psychiatry in Vietnam: From Confidence to Dismay* (Westport, CT: Greenwood Press, 1988), 1.

[122] William Date and Arnold W. Johnson, Jr., *Psychotropic Prescription Medication in Vietnam* (Alexandria, VA: Defense Technical Information Center, 1981), 1-7.

[123] Jones, 84.

[124] Camp, 1.

gap became evident, starting with the downsizing of mental health capacity in theater and the lack of veteran assistance back in the United States.[125]

The last perceived cause of combat stress emerged from the soldier personally. The meaning of combat for each individual who fought was different, but there were common shared experiences derived from unstructured and often chaotic nature of this war.[126] Unlike previous American military efforts, the Vietnam experience frequently included killing of women, children, and elderly who sometimes were the enemy, and sometimes were not.[127] Guilt rose among some military members and left them struggling to comprehend the actions they were ordered to execute. With an individual rotation schedule, unit leadership and cohesion was hindered and soldiers were often left to cope with the stresses of combat and the return home alone.

Vietnam veterans faced war abroad and were given a negative stigma by U.S. citizens upon their return to the United States. "In no prior war fought by the United States has the actual combat experience of our fighting men been less understood by the government in Washington or the public than that in the Vietnam War."[128] Citizens' disapproval of service members and the government fueled soldiers' thoughts of shame, helplessness, anger, guilt, and abandonment.[129] Although initial efforts to address combat stress on the battlefield were considered a success, the Vietnam experience is often considered a "black cloud" in American military efforts when it comes to the prevalence, detection, and prevention of PTSD.

---

[125] Camp, 6.

[126] Jones, 87.

[127] Hendis and Hass, 232.

[128] Hendis and Hass, 223.

[129] S.W.Edmendson and D. J. Platner, "Psychiatric Referrals from Khe Sanh During Siege," *U.S. Army Vietnam Medical Bulletin* (July/August 1968): 45.

Criteria Analysis of Combat Stress

Leader collaboration to address PTSD is evident. The historical experience of the United States in Vietnam reveals leaders on the battlefield collaborating early on in the war. Ground commanders and mental health providers embedded mental health capabilities in the maneuver formations and provided combat health hospitals throughout Vietnam. For example, medical units such as the 95th Evacuation Hospital and 67th Medical Group were spread throughout the country of Vietnam from 1968-1974. In 1968, the 95th Evacuation Hospital established a 320-bed hospital near the South China Sea next to the Marble Mountains. The hospital's capability included neurology, psychiatric consultations, and counseling. From the hospitals, mental health providers conducted rotational mental health assessments of units in smaller camps in the Northern Military Combat Region.[130] In 1968, the 67th Medical Group established eight hospitals, and twenty-five combat stress teams to augment units operating in the Bien Hoa, Da Nang, and Tuy Hoa regions. The teams provided combat stress care to battalion level organizations by bolstering the organic medical aid stations of the maneuver forces. The teams provided the capability of mental health treatment from point of injury and were able to link into the hospitals in the region.[131]

The evidence of leaders and followers developing a relationship to address PTSD is ambiguous in the experience of Vietnam. The bond between leader and follower was undermined from the beginning of the conflict. Most important to the leader and follower relationship was time to interact with each other to form a trusting bond.[132] The frequent rotation of soldiers was blamed for creating problems in the unit effectiveness and cohesion. Every soldier knew the exact date of expected return from overseas (DEROS). The idea that one did not have to die to come

---

[130] "Medical units where women served during the Vietnam War" Civilian Account Report Online, http://www.illyria.com/evacs.html#medcaps (accessed April 11, 2011).

[131] Ibid.

[132] Northouse, 17.

home raised hopes in soldiers. However, the rotational schedule created a constant flow of soldiers in and out of units, limiting cohesion within the unit.[133] Command positions were subject to frequent rotation. "Condensed command tours resulted in periods of poor leadership, precipitating concomitant fears in enlisted personnel that they would pay the price in blood."[134] Some commanders switched commands after three months, so it was common for a soldier to have three different company commanders and battalion commanders, each pursuing their own take on what should take place in day to day operations. For example, the 4th Infantry Division arrived in Vietnam in September 1966.[135] By mid-1967 the division was divided, conducting Operation MacArthur in Kontum Province and Operation Junction City. Three months later, most soldiers in 1st and 3rd Brigades were re-assigned to the 25th Infantry Division until individual DEROS dates arrived. When their enlistment time expired, they were re-assigned back to 3rd Brigade, 4th Infantry Division, and redeployed back to the United States. Shifting of soldiers from one unit to another limited the bond between leaders, leaders and followers, and subordinated that was needed to address problems of combat fatigue.

Field Manual 3-0, Operations states, "Every leader shoulders the responsibility that their subordinates return from a campaign not only as good soldiers, but also as good citizens with pride in their service to the Nation." [136] In part, this observation extends from the Army's experience with individual rotational policy during Vietnam. However, in the Vietnam War leaders could not shoulder this responsibility due to the rate of individual rotations, personnel shifting from unit to units, and frequent change of commands. Personnel of all ranks redeployed

---

[133] Marlowe, 3.

[134] Helmus and Glenn, 18.

[135] "Vietnam War Battalions, Brigades, Corps, Divisions, Organizations, Platoons, Units" Civilian Personnel On-Line, http://www.vietnamwar.net/organizations.htm (accessed April 12, 2011).

[136] FM 3-0, 1-20.

back to the United States alone and, in some cases, soldiers faced the effects of combat stress without any support from those who shared their experiences.

Evidence of social change was visible in the three branches of government and the armed services. Three dominant groups influenced changes for the Vietnam veterans and their mental health needs: the public, the medical doctor, and government officials elected after the war. First, public recognition of the mental health problems of veterans led to the "definition, public awareness, medical treatment, and legal use of PTSD."[137] Several groups for and against the war were developed and advocated for a nationwide network of Veteran Centers to support soldiers problems. Veterans became elected officials in all three branches of government. For example, Max Cleland, a disabled veteran, became the Director of the Veterans Administration in 1976. Senate and House of Representative committee's legislated for readjustment counseling for all veterans, and in 1979, President Carter signed Public Law 96-22 to establish Veteran Outreach programs across the nation.

Even with the availability and accessibility of programs, the military still had problems with mental health issues. "Veteran activism was directly responsible for the inclusion of PTSD in the DSM-III (Diagnostic and Statistical Manual of Mental Disorders), and was a significant influencer for the development of mental health and abuse programs in the military."[138] During the war, more than 470,000 male veterans (15.2%) and 610 female veterans (8.1%) returning from Vietnam veterans were diagnosed with combat stress.[139] A relationship between PTSD and suicide emerged from veteran case studies.[140] Within five years after the Vietnam War (and the

---

[137] Jones, 91.

[138] Jones, 97.

[139] Matthew Tull, "Rates of PTSD in Veterans" July 22, 2009, http://ptsd.about/com/od/prevalence/a/militaryPTSD.htm, (accessed December 12, 2010).

[140] Nidiffer and Leach, 23.

admission of the term PTSD into the DMS-III), mortalities studies by the Center for Disease

Control indicated 9,000 Vietnam veterans committed suicide within five years of being

discharged from service.[141]

In light of these studies, the military recognized the need to change as an organization.

The transformation to a professional force took decades to generate. Lieutenant Colonel Suzanne

Neilsen posited,

> The transformation of the U.S. Army as it went from being an institution in
> distress in the late 1960s and early 1970s during the Vietnam War, to being an
> organization that demonstrated tactical and operational excellence in the 1991
> Persian Gulf War was due to integrated reformed in personnel policy,
> organization, doctrine, training, and equipment modernization.[142]

The Vietnam War, unfortunately, set the stage for mass improvement within the organization

through all levels of the military.

The Vietnam historical experience demonstrated the effects of mental health in military

organizations. Evidence of leadership collaboration, leaders and followers addressing PTSD and

evidence of social change in the historical experience resulted in the following assessment:

	Criteria 1: Leader Collaboration	Criteria 2: Leader/Follower Relationship	Criteria 3: Social Change in the Army
Vietnam War	E	A	E

Figure 3: Summary Chart of Historical Experience #3.

Figure 3 presents an evident (E), non-evident (NE), or ambiguous (A) summary chart of

Case Study #3 to provide evidence to support the evaluation criteria. Evident (E) is favorable,

---

[141] Tull, 2009.

[142] Suzanne Neilsen, An Army Transformed: The U.S. Army's Post-Vietnam Recovery and the Dynamics of Change in Military Organizations, Strategic Studies Institute, (Carlisle Barracks, PA: U.S. Army War College, September 2010), iii.

ambiguous (A) represents null evidence, and non-evident (NE) is no evidence to support the criterion.

At first, the correlation between units conducting missions and mental health capability seemed to address the effects of combat stress on the battlefield. But soon it became apparent that what truly emerged was a phenomenon involving soldiers and combat, and a lack of leader collaboration as a means to address combat stress became obvious. The drastic increase of combat stress cases during the drawdown period dismayed political, military, and medical leaders.

Additionally, the one year deployment structure and shifting of personnel hindered the ability for leaders and followers to address PTSD within the formation. Soldiers were assigned individually and were unable to develop trust with their leadership. Leaders changed units and new causes of PTSD were studied, but it was not until the skeptical public and veterans influenced the government to change that social evolution took place. Federal programs became available to veterans and the military assumed responsibility of the harsh lessons of the war and began to rebuild.

Summary of Analysis

As demonstrated, military leaders and societal responses to men and women impaired by trauma such as PTSD occur throughout twentieth century American history.[143] World War I, World War II, and Vietnam provide historical experiences that illustrate how American military leadership encountered PTSD, or one of its predecessors, on a large scale. The American experience in World War I began with a baseline understanding of war neurosis by observing and working with the British military. Dr. Salmon established multi-echelon treatment facilities,

---

[143] Nidiffer and Leach, 13.

which increased the ability for providers to gain knowledge of war neurosis and for patients to seek treatment and return to duty. As the United States entered World War II, military leaders were determined to reduce psychiatric losses of the scale suffered in the previous World War. The military relied on personnel screening as a discriminator for service and believed that soldier selection would serve as the solution to mental health problems.[144] However, by August 1942, screening methods had proved unreliable, and war neurosis was high as hospitals were once again overrun with mental health cases. Eventually, the work of Dr. Hanson and Dr. Tureen re-invented Dr. Salmon's echeloning medical care forward throughout Allied operating lines and accepted universal susceptibility of the problem. The Army instituted change by re-naming the illness to combat exhaustion in an effort to remove stigma associated with mental health issues and present a cure to the problem.

In Vietnam, combat stress again affected military organizations. The implementation of an aggressive echeloning of care allowed in-combat combat stress levels to remain low and seemed to indicate success. However, as years of war continued, combat stress cases emerged, frequently far removed from the battlefield. The greatest increase in combat stress cases was from 1969-1971 as American forces transitioned to less intense combat operations. A new epidemic of delayed stress response surfaced in the military and leaders were once again left with an emerging problem during operations.

---

[144] Sullivan, 1964.

As evident in the criteria analysis towards each historical experience, the following assessment was accumulated:

	Criteria 1: Leader Collaboration	Criteria 2: Leader/Follower Relationship	Criteria 3: Social Change in the Army
World War I	E	A	E
World War II	E	A	E
Vietnam	E	A	E

Figure 4: Summary Chart of Historical Experience #1-3.

Figure 4 presents an evident (E), non-evident (NE), or ambiguous (A) summary chart of Case Study #1 to provide evidence to support the evaluation criteria. Evident (E) is favorable, ambiguous (A) represents null evidence, and non-evident (NE) is no evidence to support the criterion.

Key findings of World War I, World War II, and Vietnam experiences indicate leader ability to identify of emerging problem during the experience, ability to answer the correct problem, and linking the developed solution seamlessly with a higher headquarters intent and subordinate action. Therefore, although the BKD model of leadership briefly mentions the importance of collaborating, the model falls short in the ability to incorporate methods to create an environment for collecting all members' solutions efficiently. Transformational leadership theory best augments the BKD model of leadership by using techniques to flatten the leadership organization such as shared vision statements, dispersed leadership roles and responsibilities, and accountability. An example is the use of multi-functional teams comprised of experts in various fields using open communication and information to solve problems such as the gap between medical treatment plans, the unit, and the soldier diagnosed with PTSD.

The World War I, World War II, and Vietnam experiences indicate shortcomings of leaders and followers working together to face PTSD within an organization. The evidence

41

suggests that leaders must experience the same conditions as the soldier in order to create a trust between them. Leaders have the responsibility to train and equip soldiers for the best chance for success. Therefore, although the BKD model of leadership briefly mentions the importance leader and follower cohesion, the model falls short in the ability to incorporate methods that ensure the relationship. The leader-member exchange theory best augments the BKD model of leadership when using techniques to inspire open dialogue between leader and subordinates such as 360 degree feedback and shared professional development experiences.

World War I, World War II, and Vietnam experiences indicate leaders forging social change within the Army as it faced the problem of PTSD. The evidence suggests providing the best solution for an unknown problem, attitudes and programs developed by the leader, and a complete solution from initiation of change through its completion are necessary to face problems such as PTSD. Therefore, although the BKD model of leadership mentions the character and competence of a leader, the model falls short in the ability to ensure the group adapts according to the situation with least risk to its members. The situational leadership theory best augments the BKD model of leadership by incorporating maturity levels and various leadership styles of its members to build the picture of the conditions that will shape the decisions the organization will make. Situational leadership theory suggests that a combination of a leader's behavior style (telling, selling, participating, delegating) and maturity (low to high level) is applied to each situation in an attempt to solve the problem within the environment. Because the BKD leadership model is hierarchal static in nature, and assumes followership from subordinates as given, situational leadership offers a range of leadership styles that can be used by the leader to find the right match toward the problem in the environment. An example is the use of one leadership style in a basic training environment and a different leadership style in a senior service school.

The findings, through the investigation of the World War I, World War II, and Vietnam historical experience, reveal that the BKD leadership model does provide initial guidance of leaders actions. The findings also suggest that the BKD leadership model would be best served if elements of transformational, leader-member exchange, and situational leadership theory were incorporated in to the concepts of the BKD leadership model, perhaps as methods and techniques for immediate use by the organization.

Recommendations and Conclusions

Investigation of the U.S. Army's Be, Know, Do leadership model as referenced in Field Manual 6-22 and analysis of leadership theory demonstrates potential areas for improvement to assist leaders with challenges. U.S. Army leadership doctrine could benefit incorporating transformational leadership theories to assist leaders with challenges such as PTSD. Three developed criteria applied to three historical case studies addressed multi-leader collaboration, the relationship between leader and follower, and the practice of leading social change. Historical experiences representing PTSD related experiences in World War I, World War II, and Vietnam revealed that incorporation of elements of transformational, leader-member exchange, and situational leadership theories into the BKD model of leadership was warranted. Specifically, in the area of organizational structure, integration of capabilities of the leader and follower, and the relationship among members would assist leaders using the BKD leadership model to face unit issues such as PTSD. Fortunately, transformational, leader-member exchange, and situational leadership theory components can augment in the BKD leadership model. Recommendations for future studies would include an investigation of other leadership theories and effects on military organizations, the effects of personnel leadership reactions towards PTSD, and effects of PTSD outside the military would continue this line of research.

The Army would best be served to incorporate elements of transformational, leader-member exchange, and situational leadership theory into the BKD leadership model theory of

43

leadership, even if organizational structure changes need to occur. Recognizing that leadership is not only with rank and position, it is often without rank and duty position that leadership can have an effect on the organization. PTSD in a military formation is nothing new, but it is growing, evolving, and not likely to disappear in the future. Leadership though the formation, in all levels of war, is the team's best chance to create social change with regard to how the Army handles PTSD, thus ensuring the long term health of the soldier.

BIBLIOGRAPHY

American Psychiatric Association. *Diagnostic and Statistical Manual of Mental Disorders.* Washington, DC: American Psychiatric Association, 1980.

Artiss, Kenneth. "Human Behavior Under Stress: From Combat to Social Psychiatry." *Military Medicine* 28 (1963): 1011-1015.

Babington, Anthony. *Shell Shock: A History of the Changing Attitudes to War Neuroses.* London: Leo Cooper, 1997.

Bass, Bernard M. "From Transactional to Transformational Leadership: Learning to Share the Vision." *Organizational Dynamics* 18 (1990): 19-31.

Bass, Bernard M., and Ronald Riggio. *Transformational Leadership.* Portland, OR: Taylor & Francis, Inc. 2005.

Boscarino, James A. "Posttraumatic Stress Disorder and Mortality among U.S. Army Veterans: 30 Years after Military Service.*" Annals of Epidemiology* 16 (2007): 248-256.

Brookfield, Shephen. *Developing Critical Thinkers.* San Francisco, CA: Jossey-Bass, 1986.

Browne, Neil, and Stewart T. Keeley *Asking the Right Questions: A Guide to Critical Thinking.* Englewood Cliffs, NY: Prentice-Hall, 1986.

Camp, Norman. *U.S. Army Psychiatry in Vietnam: From Confidence to Dismay.* Westport: Greenwood Press, 1988.

Campbell, David and Dardis, James. "The "Be, Know, Do" Model of Leader Development." HR. Human Resources Planning (2004): 1-27.

Civilian Account Report On-Line. "Medical Units Where Women Served During the Vietnam War." http://www.illyria.com/evacs.html#medcaps (accessed April 11, 2011).

Civilian Account Report On-Line. "Vietnam War Battalions, Brigades, Corps, Divisions, Organizations, Platoons, Units." http://www.vietnamwar.net/organizations.htm (accessed April 12, 2011).

Collins, Jim. *Good to Great. Why Some Companies Make the Leap…and Other's Don't.* New York: Harper Business, 2001.

Coleman, Jules, V. *Division Psychiatry in the Southwest Pacific Area.* The History of Neuropsychiatry in the World War II, edited by W. Mullins. Washington DC: Government Printing Office, 1978.

Date, William E. and Arnold W. Johnson, Jr. *Psychotropic Prescription Medication in Vietnam.* Alexandria: Defense Technical Information Center, 1981.

Davidson, Paul. *Vietnam at War*. New York: Oxford University Press, 1991.

Dean, Eric T. *Shook over Hell: Post-traumatic Stress, Vietnam and the Civil War.*
    Cambridge: Harvard University Press, 1999.

Del Jones, Franklin and Arnold Johnson. "Medical and Psychiatric Treatment Policy and Practice
    in Vietnam." *Journal of Social Sciences* 31 (1975): 49-65.

Drayer, C.S. and A.J. Glass. *Introduction*. Medical Department, United States Army,
    Neuropsychiatry in World War II. Washington, DC: Office of the Surgeon General,
    1973.

Edmendon, S.W. and D.J. Plattner. "Psychiatric Referrals from Khe Sahn During Seige." *U.S.
    Army Vietnam Bulletin* (1968): 43-47.

Friedman, Matthew J. *Posttraumatic Stress Disorder: An Overview*. National Center for
    PTSD, July, 2010.

Gilbert, Martin. *The First World War: A Complete History*. New York: Henry Holt and
    Company, 1994.

Ginzberg, Eli. *The Lost Divisions*. New York: Columbia University Press, 1959.

Glass, A.J. *Lessons Learned*. The History of Neuropsychiatry in World War II, edited by W.
    Mullins. Washington, DC: Government Printing Office, 1978.

Haycock, Robert D. "A Time for Change: Attacking the Stressors Vice the Symptoms."
    Monograph, U.S. Army Command and General Staff College, 2009.

Hendin, Herbert and Ann Pollinger Hass. *Wounds of War*. New York: Basic Books, 1984.

Hersey, Paul and Kenneth Blanchard. *Management of Organizational Behavior: Utilizing Human
    Resources*. Englewood Cliffs, NJ: Prentice Hall, 1982.

Helmus, Todd and Russell Glenn. "Steeling the Mind: Combat Stress Reactions and Their
    Implications for Urban Warfare." Monograph, U.S. Army Command and General Staff
    College, 2005.

Jones, Barbara. "Post Traumatic Stress Disorder in the United States Legal Culture: An Historical
    Perspective from World War I through the Vietnam Conflict." Ph.D diss., University of
    Minnesota, 1995.

Jones, Edgar, Nicola Fear, and Simon Wesley. "Shell Shock and Mild Traumatic Brain Injury: A
    Historical Review." *AM Psychiatry* 164:11 (2007):1641.

Jones, Franklin. "Traditional Warfare Combat Stress Casualties." *War Psychiatry* (1995): 35-61.

Kobrin, Nancy H. and Jerry L. Kobrin, "J.M. da Costa M.D. – An
    American Civil War Converso Physician." *Shofar* 18 (1999): 1-18.

Leed, Eric J. *No Man's Land: Combat and Identity in World War I.* Cambridge: Cambridge University Press, 1981.

Liddell Hart, B.H., *Great Captains Unveiled.* Boston: Little Brown Company, 1927.

Lussier, Robert and Christopher Achua. *Leadership: Theory, Application, and Skill Development.* Ohio: Southwestern, 2009.

Macdonald, Lyn. *1915, The Death of Innocence.* New York: Henry Holt and Company, 1995.

Mannarelli, Thomas. "According for Leadership: Charismatic, Transformational Leadership Through Reflection and Self-Awareness." *Accountancy Ireland* 38 (2006): 46-48.

Marlow, D.H. "Delayed and Immediate Onset of Post Traumatic Stress Disorder." *Social Psychiatry and Psychiatric Epidemiology* (1991): 1-7.

Marx, Brian, P. "Posttraumatic Stress Disorder and Operating Enduring Freedom and Iraqi Freedom: Progress in a Time of Controversy." *Clinical Psychology Review* 29 (2009): 671-673.

Mintzberg, Henry. The Rise and Fa`ll of Strategic Planning. New York: The Free Press, 1994.

Moore, Harold and Joseph Galloway, *We Were Soldiers Once…and Young.* New York: Random House, 1992.

Neilsen, Suzanne. *An Army Transformed: The U.S. Army's Post-Vietnam Recovery and the Dynamics of Change in Military Organization.* Strategic Studies Institute. Carlisle Barracks, PA: U.S. Army War College, September 2010.

Nidiffer, F. Don and Spencer Leach. "To Hell and Back: Evolution of Combat-related Post Traumatic Stress Disorder." *Developments of Mental Health Law* 29 (2010): 1-23.

Northouse, Peter, G. *Leadership: Theory and Practice.* Thousand Oaks: Sage, 2007.

Nye, Ella C. "Specific Symptoms Predict Suicidal Ideation in Vietnam Combat Veterans with Chronic Post-traumatic Stress Disorder." *Military Medicine* 172 (2007): 1144-1147.

Oelofse, Eriaan. "Core and Peripheral Cultural Values and Their Relationship to Transformational Leadership Attributes of South African Managers." Ph.D. diss., University of Pretoria, 2006.

Pershing, John. *Final Report, Commander-In-Chief American Expeditionary Forces.* Washington: Government Printing Office, 1920.

Rejai, Mustafa and Phillips, Key. *Leaders and Leadership: An Appraisal of Theory and Research.* Westport: Praeger, 1997.

Ross, Davis. *Preparing for Ulysses: Politics and Veterans During World War II.* New York: Columbia University Press, 1969.

Shaffer, Ronald. *The Treatment of Shell Shock Cases in the AEF: A Microcosm of the War Welfare State.* America in the Great War: The Rise of the Welfare State. New York: Oxford University Press, 1991.

Shephard, Ben. "Shell Shock on the Somme." *RUSI Journal* (1996): 51-56.

Simkin, John. "The Medical Treatment of Shell Shock." http://www.spartacus.schoolnet.co.uk/ (accessed October 1, 2010).

Smythe, Donald. *Pershing: Generals in the Armies.* Bloomington, IN: Indiana University Press, 1986.

Spector, Ronald H. *After Tet.* New York: The Free Press, 1993.

Spiegel, Herbert X. "Preventive Psychiatry with Combat Troops." *American Journal of Psychiatry* 101 (November 1944): 311-312.

Sullivan, Harry S."Psychiatry and the National Defense" in *The Fusion of Psychiatry and Social Science* edited by Harry S. Sullivan, New York: Norton, 1964.

Swank, Roy and Walter Marchland. " Combat Neuroses.' *Archives of Neurology and Psychiatry* 55 (1946): 207-218.

Tull, Matthew. "Rates of PTSD in Veterans." http://ptsd.about/com/od/prevalence (accessed December 12, 2010).

U.S. Department of the Army. *FM 22-100 Military Leadership.* Washington, DC: Government Printing Office, October, 1983.

U.S. Department of the Army. *FM 3.0 Operations.* Washington, DC: Government Printing Office, December, 2001.

U.S. Department of the Army. *FM 6-22: Army Leadership.* Washington, DC: Government Printing Office, December, 2006.

U.S. Department of the Army. *Field Service Regulations.* Washington DC: Government Printing Office, 1923.

U.S. Department of the Army. *Field Service Regulations 40-34.* Washington DC: Government Printing Office, 1966.

Ward, Harry. M. *Washington's Enforcers: Policing the Continental Army.* Carbondale, IL: Southern Illinois University Press, 2006.

Yukl, Gary. *Leadership in Organizations.* Uppersaddle River, NJ: Prentice Hall, 2002.